"What a concept: a book about clinical communication skills, created by an actual skilled communication professional with way too much healthcare drama in her life! And she knows how to teach it as concrete skills, not just theory.

Transformation is always kindled by stories that make you think "We can do better." But then you have to answer, "So how do I do this?" **Patient Speak** is a masterful mix of all those dimensions, in a friendly, accessible style with a clear, easy-to-reference layout."

— **Dave deBronkart, Stage IV Cancer Survivor and Engagement Evangelist**

"Too often we look at "soft skills" as being insignificant compared to the work of medically treating patients. Nancy reminds us in **Patient Speak** that the verbal and non-verbal interactions healthcare providors have with patients have a tremendous impact in not only how satisfied and content they are but those same interactions can actually enhance or harm their care and outcomes."

— **Fred Fishback, President, Javelin Learning Solutions**

"My work focuses on what works for people on their journey towards best health. Our journey depends on the relationships among all members of our health team. Relationships rely on responsive communication. I have little energy to teach my team unless I feel fairly well. Our time is now. Let's use it well. Nancy Michael's **Patient Speak, 7 Communication Practices** provides a concise guide to share with your clinician team members. Keep a spare on hand to share."

— **Danny van Leeuwen, Opa, RN, MPH, @ Health Hats**

"**Patient Speak** offers a personal and intimate account of what it's like to be a patient and the importance of how and what things are said to us as patients. I feel honored to call Nancy a friend and colleague in our desire to improve the patient experience."

— **Kistein Monkhouse, MPA, founder of Patient Orator**

"The manner in which we address our patients and their family members can often be overlooked or not thought as significant when it comes to patient care. Nancy makes clear that words and body language have a significant impact on a patient's mental and emotional wellbeing in **Patient Speak** and provides key examples of how we can implement these concepts to up our practice of delivering quality medical care."

— **Robin Wyatt, Patient- and Family-Centered Care Advocate**

PATIENT
Speak

7 Communication Practices
To Improve Patient and Family Experience

A GUIDE FOR HEALTHCARE
PROFESSIONALS

NANCY MICHAELS

Published by Powers Press

ISBN-13: 978-1732560505

ISBN-10: 1732560501

CreateSpace Independent Publishing Platform
North Charleston, SC

Table of Contents

Patient Speak

Preface

A doctor or nurse taking the time to offer a kind word, an encouraging remark, smile, or give a fist bump to their patient, is a powerful gift that shows true compassion. It might seem like nothing, but simply being present with a patient is a present. However, many healthcare professionals seem to have forgotten the art of effective verbal and nonverbal communication—especially when interacting with patients and their family members.

The decision to choose a physician or hospital is typically based on the reputation of the doctor or hospital that resonates with us. We purchase health services like products, based on the trust and belief we have in their ability to come through for us. Quite often, it's our primary care provider (PCP) who makes the call. This was the case in my situation because of the emergency nature of my illness, which was sudden onset liver failure in 2005.

I've always worked professionally as a communicator, and my experience as an ICU patient, and my ongoing recovery, made it very clear where my skills are now needed most. My mission and purpose is to teach current and future healthcare providers on ways to more effectively communicate with patients and family members. The best way I know how to do this is to provide them with the patient's and family's perspective.

I believe that more effective communication among hospitals, physicians, technicians, and nurses, and with patients and family members, is a win-win-win situation. When patients feel they have open and honest lines of communication with their physicians and healthcare systems, I suspect that hospital stays are shorter, readmissions go down and more patients report they are more satisfied and content with their overall experience. More satisfied patients and family members become walking billboards for the amazing work hospitals, physicians, technicians, and nurses do. In the unfortunate cases where mistakes are made, patients have greater forgiveness and compassion for the practitioners and their humanity. Saving millions of dollars for everyone involved in all these positive outcomes is icing on the cake.

In 1976, Warner Slack, MD (1933–2018) at Harvard Medical School wrote that "the largest and least utilized healthcare resource is the patient him/herself." After spending nearly a decade studying computer-mediated patient interviewing, Dr. Slack concluded that patients, as the primary source of their own health information, should be encouraged to provide that information directly to their medical team to improve the quality of their own care. Communication is a two-way street and although this book is primarily written for medical professionals to become better communicators with patients and family members, a critical component of communication is in our ability to listen. Patients and family members have a lot to say and share about how we are feeling and should be used as a valuable resource as Dr. Slack suggests.

What you say and how you say it have a significant impact on your patients and their ability to heal emotionally, mentally and physically. It is my hope that **Patient Speak** provides you with a greater awareness of the power of words and actions, and the appropriate communication skills to use when treating the most critically ill to the mildly afflicted, along with their family and friends who care for and love them.

Patient Speak

About the Book

Patient Speak: 7 Communication Practices to Improve Patient and Family Experience

Patient Speak is a reference guide of communication techniques and approaches recommended for healthcare and medical professionals to use when interacting with their patient, so their patient and family members can feel the genuine concern the medical team has about the patient's overall emotional, psychological, and physical health.

Patient Speak outlines more than seventy patient-centric ways of communicating that are meaningful to patients and family members. Each of these ideas takes very little time, and costs virtually nothing.

Patient Speak helps reinforce effective communication practices that leave patients with more positive impressions about their time in a hospital. Patients have many memories of being hospitalized or very ill. However, as their health returns, the memories that remain strongest are how the medical staff and their caretakers communicated with them. Creating positive associations through thoughtful communication enhances relationships of all kinds but has an even greater effect with patients. The care and connection you have with your patients and their families, providing respect, dignity, and concern for their emotional and mental well-being, in addition to their physical needs, can be life changing.

And for that, your patients will thank you.

Patient Speak is the perfect gift to offer to colleagues during Nurse Appreciation Week or Hospital Week or other memorable occasions when medical professionals are being honored and thanked for their immense service.

To order additional copies of this book for your team, hospital, pharmaceutical company, or medical device salesforce, please contact Team@NancyMichaels.com and discover options for bulk pricing and customization.

To sign up for my 10 Keys to More Effective Patient Care go to www.NancyMichaels.com

Acknowledgments

There are so many people one needs to recognize when writing and publishing a book, it's difficult to know where to begin.

To start, I need to thank the amazing medical team I had and continue to have at Beth Israel Deaconess Medical Center starting with Dr. Michael Curry, my liver doctor who, I was told, made the call to go forward and offer me a liver transplant against all odds. To my nurse practitioner, Erin Sexton, who was with me from day one and whom I continue to see and reach out to with a question or concern to this day. To Frank Caparelli, my nurse in ICU, who took the time and had the compassion to take me outside into the sun at the loading docks of BIDMC that hot August day in 2005. To the intern who discovered that my constant nausea was caused by an inner ear imbalance and simply put a scopolamine patch behind my ear, and within twenty-four hours, I was eating without nausea for the first time in months.

My assistant, confidante and "grace under pressure" Mireia Carpio, who keeps all things running smoothly in my business (and sometimes life)! Special thanks to Cindy Murphy who has offered her creative talent on the book cover and interior layout – and has the patience of a saint. Martha Bullen has been a bevy of solid advice on this project as well as Debra Englander who gave sage guidance and helped me make wonderful professional connections. Diane Darling for her encouragement and last-minute read-throughs as well.

To my parents, who opened their hearts and home to me and my children during my illness, who spent endless hours in waiting rooms, driving from central Massachusetts to Boston to either see me or take me to yet another series of doctors' appointments or tests. To my brothers, Tom, David, and Peter, and their wives, Darlene, Lisa, and Melissa, who did whatever they could to help my parents help me, allowing my children into their homes at a moment's notice. Each and every one of them contributed to my recovery. They helped with my care, medications, and overall mental state with their kind actions and words. To my three children, Chloe, Noah, and Sophie, who lived through this terrifying time for young children, and who were only nine, seven, and six at the time. I'm forever in debt to my family for their selflessness, love, and care for me and my children during this most challenging time in our lives.

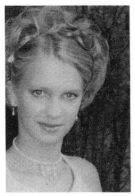

Erica Stewart Mullins
(1984 – 2005)

Finally, to my organ donor, Erica Stewart Mullins, who lost her life too soon, at age twenty-one, with two beautiful babies left behind. There are no words to thank someone I've never known whom I now carry inside me. The gift of life from organ donation is the greatest gift I've ever been given. Please, if you haven't registered to be an organ donor, do so at your local registry of motor vehicles or go to www.donatelife.net/facts.

I've had three remarkable experiences that have allowed me to see firsthand how interconnected we all really are. The first two were the adoptions of my two daughters, and the third was to have been an organ recipient. Never underestimate the goodness and kindness of strangers. I have been given the greatest gifts of all from people I have never met.

How fortunate am I?

Patient Speak

Introduction

It Sucks to Be Sick

Let's face it—it's no fun to be a patient. Trust me, I know.

It's probably not a lot of fun to be a caregiver of a patient either. I've had little firsthand experience at this, and when I have, it has not been easy. Unfortunately, I know there will be plenty of opportunity to learn as I and the loved ones around me age.

No one said it better than Rosalyn Carter when she said this about caregivers:

"There are only four kinds of people in the world:
Those who have been caregivers,
Those who are currently caregivers,
Those who will be caregivers,
and those who will need caregivers."

I can appreciate these sentiments even more now than I did when I first became a parent and my children had health challenges. My daughter had eczema and my son was diagnosed on the autism spectrum. I got a bigger dose of needing caretakers when I fell ill in 2005.

Patient Speak was written primarily for professional caretakers, providers of medical services such as nurses, doctors, physical therapists, radiology technicians, and phlebotomists, but also applies to personal caregivers as well. You have devoted a portion of your personal and/or professional life to helping to treat and heal the ill. I'm so personally grateful and thankful for your dedication, especially to all of you who cared for me when I was ill. Without you, I would not have made it out alive, and I will never forget the kindness, compassion, and care you bestowed upon me.

Patient Speak: 7 Communication Practices to Improve Patient and Family Experience, is a call to look at patients as individual human beings with lives and struggles of their own prior to or during their illness. This book was written to be a guide and gentle reminder of the amazing power you, as healthcare providers, have in the verbal and nonverbal interactions with your patients and their families. It is also applicable to the interactions you have with your coworkers. My desire is to provide you with patients' perspectives, to uncover their opinions, attitudes, beliefs, feelings, and emotions around the care they receive, and the profound effect your communication has on their well-being.

May you take something away from the personal stories and examples provided in this book, and pledge to listen to and actually hear the viewpoints and voices of your patients and their family members in your current and future interactions.

Patient Speak

Chapter 1

To Your Health

*"When you have your health, you have everything.
When you do not have your health, nothing matters at all."*

— Augusten Burroughs, Author

I never realized how true this saying was until I first got sick thirteen years ago. Up to that point, I had been a very vibrant and strong person. This cliché is heard all too often but is rarely said by a young, physically, and mentally well person like me. According to Ralph Waldo Emerson, "The first wealth is health." So true; however, it is often something we take for granted...but only when we are healthy. Most of us realize how fortunate we are to be well only after illness strikes us or a loved one.

I lived a very healthy and full life until age forty-one, when I found myself in the midst of a marital separation, raising three young children aged six, seven, and nine, managing a large house on nearly three acres of land, and running my speaking and consulting business where travel was a weekly event. To say stress got the better of me is an understatement.

After being unable to walk off a plane after giving a speech in Atlantic City, New Jersey, I was taken to my local ER where I was then transported to the ICU at a major Boston medical facility. I was told in short order that I was undergoing complete organ failure. My kidneys improved, but my liver would need to be replaced. It was a surreal experience to hear those words and take that information in. Almost unbelievable. I had been an organ donor; the thought of being an organ recipient was a foreign concept to me, until then.

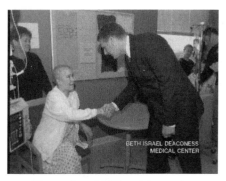

November 2005 – six months after my transplant surgery and subsequent brain surgery

After the operation, I remained in a coma for two months. When I awoke, I had a trachea intubation that I needed to be weaned off of during the next month before going to rehab for six weeks. Post rehabilitation, I was then readmitted to Beth Israel Deaconess Medical Center (BIDMC) with a "failure to thrive" diagnosis, typically given to preemies or end-of-life patients. I remained there for six weeks before being released, only to return eleven more times during the next six months for various complications (e.g., rejection episodes, high potassium blood levels, aspergillum in my lungs, etc.).

I then had to move in with my parents (away from my children and home) for the following six months. In the meantime, I lost legal and physical custody of my children, which took a year and a half and thousands of dollars in legal fees to regain.

There were days that I was absolutely despondent and suicidal, overcome with grief and emotions. I remember one day lying on the couch crying to my dad—he was not known for his diplomacy—who had this reaction. "Nancy, your only job right now is to get better because if you don't do that, you'll never have the things you're wanting now." Nice. I was outraged that my father could be so insensitive to my plight and my need for empathy and understanding. I was angry and really upset for at least seventy-two hours.

I then began to think of the smallest things I could be grateful for. I started off slowly. I was grateful that no one was depending on me to do anything for them. I was grateful my mom was feeding me and my children when they visited. I was grateful I could sleep without worry or guilt. Little statements of gratitude became big ones and I began to realize my father's words were correct. Without my health, I truly had nothing. I could achieve none of this without the gift of gratitude. Baby steps.

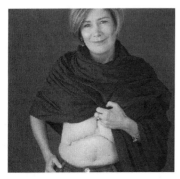

2007, almost two years after my liver transplant

My experiences as a patient in ICU for six consecutive months, rehabilitation, and a return trip to the hospital, make me uniquely qualified to offer some useful advice for medical professionals. My twenty-plus years of experience as a business consultant and public speaker, before and after my illness, complete a trifecta of experiences that allow me to see this issue from many sides.

As I reflect on my healthcare interactions, I have come up with key communication techniques that can help improve patients' experiences and increase patient satisfaction, overall outcomes, and safety. The concept of treating others as we wish to be treated is simple, and it will take work, training and self-discipline to be implemented. This book will outline some communication strategies that I hope will inspire you, and help you understand that even small changes can make a big impact in the way a patient hears or interprets what they are told. I want to help medical professionals deliver a positive experience for the patient, *regardless* of what is said, because it is more often *how* something is said that makes the biggest difference.

Here's the good news: as a member of three patient and family advisory councils, a speaker at many industry patient-centric conferences, and a patient experience consultant to healthcare providers, I know that work is being done to truly listen to patients about ways to improve our complex healthcare system. It is my hope that you help continue the practice of clear and compassionate communication, with your peers and patients.

It's taken me thirteen years to get to the point where I could share this message, to help health professionals see things through the eyes of a patient, and to inspire individuals and family members in a health crisis or feeling ill.

I'm ready now.

Patient Speak

Chapter 2

The Case for More Effective Communication in Medical Settings

"We have two ears and one mouth so that we can listen twice as much as we speak."

— Epictetus, Philosopher

I sought out a career in communication. I achieved my undergrad and graduate degrees in communication (Emerson College). I became a publicist in Boston, working for a public relations and advertising firm and a Boston network affiliate TV station. I then ran my own business as a consultant to smaller companies that needed marketing and PR assistance.

From there, I began authoring books on and speaking about business development and communicating a clear message to specific customer bases. I am not a physician, nurse, radiologist, hospital CEO, or medical provider, and I don't claim to be any of those things. However, with my background in communications, I can help teach you how to be a more effective communicator with your patients, their family members, and your coworkers.

Except for a class or two during medical school, students historically have not been taught the importance of how to provide information to patients and family members with credibility, compassion, and clarity. The art of learning effective listening skills has also not been in the curriculum. Only recently have medical schools taught their students that they need to be very mindful of patient satisfaction, and how it affects patient survey scores.

As you probably know, HCAHPS *(Hospital Consumer Assessment of Healthcare Providers and Systems)* is a patient satisfaction survey for adult inpatients that is required by CMS (the Center for Medicare and Medicaid Services) for all hospitals in the United States. The scores are used to calculate incentive payments for hospital reimbursement. Under the value-based purchasing program, hospitals can be penalized for low HCAHPS scores.

Therefore, viewing patients as consumers is a trend that will continue to gain popularity and priority among hospitals, healthcare systems, and providers. So, how will these concepts of patient satisfaction and experience be taught to medical students?

According to a 2015 report from *STAT*, an online national publication from Boston Globe Media Partners that covers health, medicine, and life sciences, "Aspiring doctors may not think they have time to gaze at paintings or play the viola while they're cramming for anatomy tests. But Harvard Medical School thinks students should be doing more of that, and the school is not alone." Harvard is helping medical students become more empathic and reflective doctors through the launch of a new initiative to use more drama, dance, and literature in their teachings. Harvard is not alone. A growing number of schools are making more direct efforts to bring the arts and humanities into educating medical students.

Visiting museums is part of the Yale School of Medicine curriculum, and analyzing paintings is used as an exercise in improving their skills at empathy and consideration. This program has been replicated at colleges and universities throughout the country, including Brown University. Narrative Medicine is being taught at Columbia where students take classes in writing, fiction, obituary writing, and the visual arts. Penn State College of Medicine is the first medical school in the country that has its own humanities department where students can take a Comics and Medicine course that fulfills a required humanities elective. Many more of these programs are being initiated in medical schools.

Clearly, all of these ways to improve patient satisfaction scores are communication based. In 2014 a *Becker Hospital Review* stated, "Improved communication increases efficiency, which translates to better service. Better service ultimately leads to higher HCAHPS scores, and that is what will separate the good from the great."

Patient Speak

In my education, work experience, writing, and speaking in public, I've learned much about how to be a more effective communicator. As a patient, I know firsthand what a difference compassionate communication made in my day-to-day existence and ultimate recovery. It made me feel like I was more than just a critically ill patient—that I was an important human being who my medical team wanted to help get better.

There are seven communication skills that I believe are necessary in life but specifically in medicine. Each of the following chapters will focus on one of these *Seven Cs:*

1. Credibility

2. Collaboration

3. Clarity

4. Context

5. Concreteness

6. Courtesy or Consideration

7. Compassion

Chapter 2: The Case for More Effective Communication

Patient Speak

Chapter 3

The First C of Communication – Credibility

"Trust is the glue of life. It's the most essential ingredient in effective communication. It's the foundational principle that holds all relationships."

— Stephen R. Covey, author, speaker, businessperson

Credibility, *adjective.*

1: capable of being believed; believable
"a credible statement;"

2: worthy of belief or confidence; trustworthy
"a credible witness."

Patient Speak

A doctor, medical practice, hospital, or healthcare system survives or thrives based on their credibility—the beliefs that people have about them, their abilities, and reputation.

Many of us (as patients) are referred to specific doctors within hospitals depending on our PCPs or specialists (in most cases), based on our current health status or treatment needs. In my case, it was my primary care physician who had seen me the week prior to going to my local ER and was called to make the decision on where I should be admitted when my blood tests revealed organ failure. My doctor had a relationship with my transplant team and had the trust and faith in them to make that referral. For that I'll be eternally grateful, given that I ultimately received a positive outcome.

Credibility and trust has to be present among medical colleagues in order to make essential referrals and to provide short and long-term solutions and treatments for patients.

As patients, we will also refer others to our physicians who we know, like, and most importantly, trust.

Although your credibility, trust, and reputation as a reputable physician or nurse can take decades to establish, it takes only one negative incident to ruin your standing and an eternity to reconstruct your position. Therefore, you must continually work to gain and retain your integrity among your patients.

Your credibility and the trust you earn are built up over time. Here are ten ways you can increase your credibility and build trust with patients right now and in the future.

1. Communicate frequently and with honesty.

This builds confidence and trust with both patients and their family members. A lack of communication creates distance and can cause a doctor/nurse and patient relationship to break down.

Make yourself as accessible as possible to your patients and their families. Provide a way for them to reach you (cell phone number, calling hours, etc.) or someone on your team if you are not available.

2. Competency reigns supreme.

We seek out medical care from the best possible sources and from those with the greatest experience. As medicine becomes more consumer-centric, patients and their family members are looking for professionals they believe to be competent. The best way to showcase your competency and to build credibility is to be consistent in your actions over time and show an ability and a willingness to receive feedback and improve.

Share new insights, findings, and so on with your patients on an ongoing basis. Being willing to answer their questions in person, by written communications, or in your daily interactions with them, are all effective ways to show your expertise and abilities, thereby enhancing your credibility.

3. Manage the patient care process.

It's important to lead the way and assure the person in your care that you are coordinating and guiding the suggested course of treatment (with patient/family input, of course).

Explain to your patients that you are aware of all the moving parts involved in their case and that you will be (in part or in whole) responsible for managing their care among many providers and are interested in their opinions and concerns. This is one of the greatest concerns that patients and their family members have—that the team is not working in unison. Demonstrate that this is true by saying so or being present when other team members are updating patients on a course of action.

4. Be a person of your word.

Say what you mean and mean what you say.

Make a promise to do the best you possibly can in caring for your patients...and keep it. It's okay to remind them of what you said and why you said it in case they forget, are fearful, or confused.

5. Become a mentor and coach by providing encouragement and hope.

Think of yourself as the navigator on their medical road map. Understand that your patients may need your reassurance at times and be willing to offer that as often and as best you can.

Offer your guidance and clear explanations of decisions, tests, and procedures to your patients. Your input can alleviate fear, create better understanding of why tests or procedures are being done, and increase your patients' belief in your expertise.

6. Rome wasn't built in a day and neither is trust.

Keep in mind that trust is built one interaction at a time. As trust is established, there is greater potential for patient compliance. Patients will often work harder, be more driven to do what's being suggested, and have a greater will to recover when the feel they are in a partnership with you for their wellbeing.

Small things make a big difference to patients. Smile when you see them, pat their hands, and make eye contact. Such nonverbal communication creates a stronger bond and greater faith in the relationship patients have with you. Express to patients what they or their family members (if applicable) need to do to meet the expectations of getting better—both yours and theirs.

7. Show patients and their families how much you care.

Take the time to "see" your patients and look at them as individual human beings.

Simply saying you're upset to see what they must be going through shows caring and compassion, and lets them know you have your patients' best interests at heart.

8. Attempt to always do the right thing.

Integrity is a big part of establishing credibility.

Explain why you think a course of treatment, action, or medication is what you believe is needed. When patients and their families know what the reasoning is behind decisions, fear and confusion dissipate.

9. If a mistake is made, admit it.

Mistakes do happen, hopefully very infrequently. However, if a gaffe occurs, it's best to admit it as soon as possible and to share the potential solution of what can and will be done to correct it or prevent it from happening again. Showing your vulnerability and humanity builds trust.

An apology and explanation of what occurred, and what steps are being taken to ensure it won't happen again, go a long way in solidifying relationships. So often, people can move on after a mistake much more easily when it is acknowledged than when it is hidden.

10. Listen and learn.

To be credible and trusted, it's best to take the time to hear your patients and their family members. Nothing can be learned from them unless you learn to truly listen.

You can facilitate learning by asking questions of your patients and truly hearing what they say. "Reflective listening" seeks to understand what your patients' ideas or thoughts are. You present their ideas back in your own words to ensure that you've understood their opinions or ideas correctly. This helps you to fully comprehend what your patients are trying to say, and often you'll learn more by listening than by talking.

Questions to Ask Your Team

What are the ways we believe we are establishing trust with our patients and family members?
- In person
- Online
- With referral sources

What is our protocol or process for introducing ourselves to patients and their family members?

How do you show that you are helping to manage the process of their experience from the doctor's office toward admission?

What are some of the ways you demonstrate good listening skills?

Patient Speak

Chapter 4

The Second C of Communication – Collaboration

"The role of a creative leader is not to have all the ideas; it's to create a culture where everyone can have ideas and feel that they're valued."

— Ken Robinson, English educator

Collaboration, *noun. verbs*
(used without an object), collaborated, collaborating

1: to work, one with another; to cooperate, as on a literary work *"they collaborated on a novel;"*

2: to cooperate, usually willingly, with an enemy nation, especially with the enemy occupying one's country *"he collaborated with the Nazis during World War II."*

Patient Speak

Collaboration is is about demonstrating mutual respect for all members of the medical team and communicating as a collective voice with patients and family members. This tone of respect is set at the top of the organization and helps to ensure that a collaborative team gets along easily, they are proactive in their communication, and team members are aware of what each of them provides across the continuum of healthcare. Patients sense and feel when tensions exist among medical team members, versus the relief they feel when they view their team as a collaborative one.

Employee engagement must be a priority within medical settings. Happy and content employees make for more satisfied patients and family members.

Coordination of care can only be achieved through collaboration and is of critical concern to patients and family members. It's a great fear among patients and caretakers that the team is not fully collaborative, and that one group may not know what the other is recommending.

My family had a doctor that met with them each day that I was first in ICU, and they were fully aware of what was going on with my case. He explained to them the course of action that would be taken by each department that was involved with my case. It was very reassuring to them to meet with "Dr. B" on an almost daily basis to get a coordinated update among all team members.

One day, my family came in and asked to speak with Dr. B and were told, "he's left and taken another job in Tennessee." My parents were devastated. For them, there was no closure in the relationship that had been built between them and Dr. B, and more importantly there was no transition between Dr. B and the other team member who would take on the role of the spokesperson for all team members as Dr. B had become to my family. They had tremendous faith in the entire team due to Dr. B's obvious knowledge and explanation of what was happening that day and what the expected course of action would be that involved all parties who were caring for me.

A better solution to this challenge would have been to have scheduled a transition meeting to inform my family of the change in contacts with Dr. B present (ideally) along with the new liaison who would fill his role. A 15-minute conversation could have improved the concern and fear my parents had in not knowing that my team's plan or objectives would be communicated to them. When Dr. B left, they no longer had a point person they could call upon who knew all of the moving parts of my case. They met individually with my doctors from that point on.

A perceived lack of collaboration or awareness amongst all medical personnel can be extremely frightening to patients and family members. It's important to always let patients and family members know that their team is working together to come up with the best possible solutions and care available. It is never wise to leave them to wonder if the medical team are communicating and working in concert with one another. There needs to be a conscious effort to take the time to explain this to patients and family members.

1. Lead by example.

The way you conduct yourself among peers and patients, showing trust and compassion, will speak volumes and is your strongest selling point. Act and assume the position of leadership regardless of your position on a team.

Acknowledge patients by their names and introduce (or reintroduce) yourself to them and their family members when you enter their rooms. Explain who you are and what your role on the team is and will be.

2. Value accountability in yourself and others.

Expect it and express it to coworkers and patients.

Share your role on the team directly with your patients. Explain what you are responsible for in their care and when you expect to see them again.

3. Celebrate diversity and teamwork.

Honor the differences among your team and let them know you respect their expertise and unique perspectives.

Share with patients publicly who each person on the team is and what each brings to the table in their healthcare plan. Your expression of confidence in the team and your verbal acknowledgment of this with your patients creates a more solid and trustworthy approach to your work and their care. One of the biggest fears among patients is that one person is unaware of what the other person is doing in their treatment and care which generates a feeling that the team is not working together. Patients become anxious when they sense this. Therefore, telling patients and their families what role each person has on the team is comforting and necessary to increase their confidence in their care.

4. Give and be receptive to feedback.

Constructive feedback is a welcome way to learn and improve. Be open to others' assessments by demonstrating your belief in your team's opinions. Strive to always be learning and open to productive dialogue with the desire to improve.

Model your own openness to feedback by asking patients or caretakers how they're feeling about what you might have just said regarding their care. You become more human and are perceived as being compassionate and trustworthy when you seek out the opinions of others.

5. Never gossip about or disparage your coworkers.

Be on guard for negative body language among your team when meeting with a patient or family member.

Patients sense tension between medical personnel, and it can make them very uncomfortable. It chips away at the confidence they have about the collective care they are receiving. Whenever possible, offer a specific compliment to a coworker in front of your patients or their family members. In large part, they will believe what you believe.

6. Approach everything with excellence.

Show people you live and work by the highest of standards. Do not ever accept less in your work or words.

Share your work ethic and approach to what you do with your patients when you talk to them by yourself as well as in front of team members. Act the way you say you will and people will believe you.

7. Be accessible to all.

People who make themselves unavailable can appear to be hiding something. Make yourself as accessible as possible.

Share with all (coworkers, patients, family members, or caretakers) when you are free to talk with them further. Providing a direct way for them to reach you or to leave a message is also reassuring and can decrease anxiety.

8. Accept responsibility.

Never blame others when things go wrong. Taking ownership when something occurs that should not have happened instills confidence, even if it was not specifically your fault.

Patient Speak

The people you work with or who are under your care will always be watching you. When and if a mistake is made on your watch, whether you are personally responsible for it or not, let a patient know that you are going to take care of it. When they know you have accepted the burden of uncovering what happened and correcting it, or ensuring it won't happen again, you solidify a relationship based on trust.

9. Bring out the best in others.

When you show interest in other team members and what they can accomplish, you make them feel important and necessary to the team.

When you do this in front of your patients, they sense your belief in the team of people who are taking care of them. This increases the confidence that they have in you, your coworkers, and the level of care they are receiving.

10. Add value in all that you do.

Make an effort to provide significant contributions that are of value to your patients.

The only way to find out what is of value to your patient is to ask them. "What can I or someone on the team do for you that would make this experience a better one for you?" Chances are they will tell you, and you will then know what "value" you are adding to that patient's experience.

Questions to Ask Your Team

How are we engaging with one another within our department or specialty group?

Are their ways we could do more to work together more effectively? How so?

Are we doing a good job sharing with patients and family members what role each team member is playing in their care?

How could we improve how we communicate with each other as well as our patients and family members about our roles across the continuum of care?

Patient Speak

Chapter 5

The Third C of Communication – Clarity

"Clarity trumps persuasion."

— Flint McLaughlin, American marketing expert

Clarity, *noun.*

1: clearness or lucidity as to perception or understanding; freedom from indistinctness or ambiguity.

2: the state or quality of being clear or transparent to the eye; translucent: *"the clarity of pure water."*

Patient Speak

The ultimate aim of communication is to speak in a way that is easily and clearly understood. Communication should be a simple, accessible, and useful conversation, that keeps the door open for further clarification if necessary.

Clear contact between medical team members is necessary to ensure that instructions are straightforward and explicit. When patients and family members are in a state of stress, confused about their case and what is being recommended or done, being clear is tantamount to the most successful outcome.

The night before my actual liver transplant, it was decided by my medical team that I might not be a candidate to be a recipient due to the severity of my situation. They were fearful I wouldn't make it through the surgery. I almost didn't. At the time, my dad was in total denial after hearing my doctors clearly state that I was being taken off the list to receive the liver transplant. My father kept asking, "but when she gets put back on the list, how long will it be until you find a liver for her?"

My other family members were very much aware of what my surgeon and medical team were saying, but somehow it was lost on my dad. After my recovery, my mom explained the conversation and was so grateful that my doctor and team were clear yet sensitive when they were delivering this devastating news. My family realized that my medical team was being very clear, and yet the news was too upsetting for my dad to hear. Thankfully for me, they made the decision within 12 hours. They opted to take the risk of providing me with a second chance at life by choosing to go forward with the transplant that happened one day after further consideration.

Always remember though that in times of chaos, clarity with compassion can help patients and families better comprehend and accept even the worst of news. Allowing patients and caretakers to have the feelings they do (denial, uncertainty, confusion or a general lack of understanding) and acknowledging them (by stating that "I know this is very upsetting news for you," or "I'm sure you were not expecting this and I realize how difficult this is for you to hear," etc.) is also valued interaction and communication between a medical team and patient or family members— despite what the news might be. Here are other ways to retain clarity in your communication with the ill, as well as their caretakers.

1. Use plain language.

It's tempting to speak in the jargon of our industry. This may not be a problem when talking to colleagues who "know" the language, but it can create barriers and confusion when we are talking to those outside of our industry, leaving individuals bewildered about what it is we are actually saying. Limit your use of vernacular, idioms, acronyms, and complex words or phrases. As long as they don't affect the accuracy of your communication or alter its meaning, replace high-level or technical lingo with common words or names whenever possible.

When explaining a course of action, prognosis, or a series of necessary tests to patients or family members, keep in mind that they did not attend medical school. Technical names of illnesses, conditions, or treatments will mean little to them and often lead to their thinking of the worst-case scenario(s) when that was never your intention. When talking to patients, talk to them with respect and in simple terms they can easily understand.

2. Speak to your target audience.

While a spoken word, phrase, or sentence may seem common to one group of individuals, it might not to another. Therefore, take into consideration and account for such factors as cultural differences, familiarity with the subject matter, language barriers, and so on.

If you sense your patient or the patient's family member is having difficulty in fully comprehending what you're saying, simply ask, "Is this making sense to you, or do you need me to clarify something?" Then listen. You might have to repeat what you said, which will make you more valuable to the people you serve. They will appreciate that you took the time to be clear and that they were treated with respect.

3. Be literal but be sensitive to the feelings of others.

Some readers have difficulty distinguishing between implied and literal meanings. Having a son on the autism spectrum has given me great insight that I didn't have before becoming his mother. My son Noah takes in his information differently. The "gray area" is often not obvious to him. When you are explaining to someone the "facts" of a situation, you might need to include a definition of a word or phrase for greater clarity.

Because patients reflect the general public in terms of unique ethnicities, learning challenges, language barriers, and so on, pay careful attention to ensure that what you're communicating is being understood. Attempting to find their "gray area" and addressing it is essential for clear communication.

4. Present your ideas in a logical order.

Before you can write in a clear style, you must arrange your thoughts in an orderly manner. This ensures your ideas will flow smoothly and build logical bridges to help patients make sense of what you are saying. The same is true when talking to someone. Setting the stage for the conversation, starting at the beginning, and offering step-by-step instructions will make your message more coherent.

As patients, when information is being presented to us, we often feel that we are drinking from a fire hose. Just as often, it's not something we are prepared to hear, and that makes the task of understanding that much more difficult. Take things slowly by stating something like, "The first thing we need to think about is..." It's important not to get too far ahead of where patients might be psychologically as well. A good rule of thumb is to present up to a maximum of three ideas, instructions, recommendations, and prognoses at a time—small steps that patients can take in and comprehend.

5. Provide practical examples where applicable.

Communicating ideas or concepts that are based on complex and abstract subject matter automatically make them a challenge to fully comprehend. Providing practical examples to help patients and their family members better understand an idea, process, event, or problem will avoid confusion.

If a patient is upset or distraught about something— an upcoming procedure, tests, or treatments—offering suggestions of how other patients have coped with this situation can help alleviate anxiety, and shows you care and understand.

6. Give alternative representations to clarify meaning when applicable.

Supplement what you say with a drawing or visual aid to help clarify the meaning of your message. Illustrations, pictures, diagrams, symbols, and other visual depictions may lead to quicker and more effective comprehension because the message is communicated in a different way.

A picture really is worth a thousand words and drafting a quick picture for your patients might help them better understand, especially if they are visual learners.

7. Truly listen and repeat what you hear for better understanding and clarity.

The most effective learning comes through listening. To be truly clear, take the time to learn from people and hear their thoughts, concerns, and fears.

Watch your patients' or family members' body language; it will provide you with clues that there may be a lack of clear understanding of what you have said or are trying to say.

8. Always be communicating.

Truly effective, clear communication involves consistently sharing information in a proactive and transparent way.

When communicating with patients—particularly those who are unable to talk—always explain to them what you are doing. Every patient wants to be "in the know," especially when they see things happening around them and are not informed of what is occurring. Explain what you are doing, or why machines are beeping, or what will happen next (when a patient needs to be ready for a test or procedure, not hours beforehand) and do so in a consistent way according to a protocol of best practices. Tell patients and family members what they need to hear and don't cover it up. Clarity always trumps persuasion.

9. Be consistent.

Be as consistent and certain as you can be when expressing your opinions or views. Changing your mind or acting uncertain (knowing that uncertainty does exist at times and may be beyond your control) can undermine your credibility. Deliver bad news and be sensitive when delivering it.

It's always important to be open and honest with patients and their families. Many times, it's the way you say something (or don't) that has a positive or negative affect on people. Your tone, body language, and clear delivery are significant. Always remember the value of providing hope, especially to patients. If they believe that there is a chance of improving, that belief has an immense impact on their emotional and psychological well-being, and patients and family members will always remember your encouragement.

10. Remove distractions.

Clarity can only come from your focused attention. Remove the distractions when talking to another person or group of people. Turn all mobile devices off and offer your undivided attention.

Patient Speak

Patients want and need your undivided attention. Emergencies do happen of course. However, being present to them without distractions when you're answering their questions or delivering new information is very important. When you give your patients your full and undivided attention, they feel your clarity and your ability to help them, they feel valued and important, and their faith in you and the process is enhanced.

Questions to Ask Your Team

Are we attempting to be clear and sensitive simultaneously to our patient's and family's feelings?

How do we do that most effectively?

Why is it important to speak in simple terms and how can we encourage our co-workers to use plain language when speaking with patients and family members?

Patient Speak

Chapter 6

The Fourth C of Communication – Context

"People have entire relationships via text message now, but I am not partial to texting. I need context, nuance and the warmth and tone that can only come from a human voice."

— Danielle Steel, American novelist

Context, *noun.*

1: the parts of a written or spoken statement that precede or follow a specific word or passage, usually influencing its meaning or effect: *"you have misinterpreted my remark because you took it out of context."*

2: the set of circumstances or facts that surround a particular event, situation, etc.

Patient Speak

Without providing *context*—the conditions or circumstances that establish the environment for your question, concept, or statement—your audience will not fully understand what you are trying to say. Context influences and improves patient comprehension. As mentioned previously in Chapter 5 on "Clarity," context relies strongly on the sequence and relationship of your sentences and the meaning you're trying to convey.

As human beings, we experience an important cognitive process in comprehending and making sense of what is being said. We connect a preceding statement with one that follows to more clearly provide us with the context of a situation. This is why thinking through what you are saying and the order in which you are saying it provides context to the listener.

A role-playing exercise between interns and patients (who were part of an ICU Patient and Family Advisory Council) practicing hospital intakes was conducted recently. The female intern asked the "patient" what her end-of-life wishes were and if she had a healthcare proxy. Both important questions to have answers to; however, the patient's feedback was that framing the questions in that way and upon her entry to the ICU would have caused her unnecessary stress and anxiety because she had no idea she was as sick as she was prior to being admitted.

When providing feedback to the intern, the patient's suggestion was to say, "Gloria (not her real name), we have to ask you questions that are sometimes uncomfortable, but we need to ask all of our patients who are admitted to the ICU. Do you mind if I go ahead and ask them of you?" That way, the patient believes (correctly) that these questions are standard operating procedure—not unique to her because of the severity of her illness. Framing the situation by putting it in context (that this is a system in place that needs to be followed) normalizes what could be a very frightening experience for a patient.

1. Manage complex situations.

Take the time to think through issues of concern. Always attempt to make what is complicated simple.

Allow patients and family members to express themselves, their concerns, and their fears about their illness or symptoms. Let them know that every case is unique, and although they may have similarities to other patients with the same diagnosis, it's important not to draw their own conclusions. Reassure them that their medical team is in communication with one another and decisions are made together, not individually.

2. Frame conversations.

Conversations or probing questions in tense situations can cause more anxiety than necessary. It's important to know and empathize with the people you're talking to and understand where they might be coming from.

It's important to set the stage of the conversations with patients and family members by letting them know that your intention is to provide an update of their situation, suggest a path that they'd like the patient or family members feedback on, and allow time for any questions. This provides a framework for the interchange and if a patient or family member knows that their opinion will be taken into consideration and their questions will be answered, they are more likely to listen to what you are saying in the moment. Sharing with them what the collective team is working on is also very comforting for both patients and family members.

3. Remove irregularities in communicating and take your time.

When behavior is consistent, it creates stability and trust. Inconsistent communication creates distrust. Do not rush when approaching a conversation with someone or when making a difficult decision. Always take the time to think things through before acting too quickly.

As in the previous example, there are many ways something can be discussed or asked of a patient in a clear, consistent, and nonthreatening context. Humans like consistency, offering a structure and sequence of communicating with a patient or family member is reassuring and familiar. Inconsistent processes within (and even outside) medical settings create anxiety and distrust. Establish protocols and systems to alleviate inconsistencies in your approach to patient care for consistent and positive outcomes.

With standards and systems in place, time is built into certain exchanges you might have with patients. When no protocol exists, or when you are questioned by patients about information you are not privileged to share or are uncertain about, it is best to hear them out and promise to return with someone who can respond to their questions or concerns.

4. Understand the concept of "previewing expectations."

This concept is used in behavioral medicine; however, its implications can be applied to anyone in any situation. Previewing expectations simply means communicating and sharing with people what they can look forward to or anticipate happening in the future. Communicating this way helps your patients put their health situation in context.

https://www.nancymichaels.com/single-post/2017/08/18/Previewing-Expectations

In patient care, this level of communication is critical to receiving compliance among patients and to fully prepare them for what is expected of them.

Likewise, overexplaining something while someone is in the hospital can be unnecessary and unproductive. Knowing when to preview expectations or not to is an art unto itself. According to most patients, there is no need for a three-hour warning of a procedure that is scheduled hours in advance or might not happen at all. When used effectively, previewing expectations helps patients to know, understand, and act on the presumption of future activities.

5. Discharge begins at intake.

Money and time can be saved with this approach to "preview expectations" and expect a more positive outcome.

This is especially effective with patient intake (when discharge expectations should begin and be explained as well). Most people do not like surprises when it comes to their health and need to know what they might need to do to prepare themselves to enter a hospital, and maybe more importantly, what they should anticipate when they go home. How can people know that they will need help (or what kind of help) when they return home if they are not told specifically what to expect? In the end, a patient who was well-informed from the beginning will be much happier and will be "expecting" the course of events to happen within a particular timeframe, barring any challenges or complications that may arise. If this is done effectively, stays could be shorter, readmissions would be less frequent, and patients and family members would be more content with the process throughout the care continuum.

https://www.nancymichaels.com/single-post/2018/08/06/ Discharge-Begins-at-Intake

6. Convey confidence when describing circumstances or situations.

Hearing and seeing people who are confident in their tone and bearing, and can back up what they are saying within the context of circumstances at hand, encourage their listeners to believe in them. When you speak to a patient or their family with conviction about the background of that particular patient's condition, their confidence in your abilities, and their optimism, increases.

Patients appreciate a confident approach to communication. It shows you believe in the suggested plan of treatment for their individual and particular care and that you stand by your recommendation. Your confidence in your communication offers a sense of certainty when things can be uncertain.

7. Be transparent when setting the stage or describing a situation or making recommendations.

When you start a conversation by openly sharing a similar situation you have experienced (or retelling another's story), you show your transparency and vulnerability. This approach quickly helps you to be viewed as a human being with feelings and real-life understanding. These qualities offer context and establish trust and believability as well.

By offering a similar example of how you, a family member, or another patient handled what your patient is experiencing, you create greater context and validity to your recommendation. Be as open and honest as possible; tell patients or family members that you want to be very clear and transparent and only share information applicable to their case. Patients appreciate this clear and rich communication more than you know.

8. Vulnerability and empathy puts their fears in context.

Connection and context is created through sharing with patients and family members. When you share your human side, express your feelings, worries, or concerns, and you empathize with them, people relate and connect to you on a personal level.

Patients feel an almost constant state of vulnerability. Their dignity is often taken from them as they have to rely on others for things they used to be able to do on their own and would never normally ask, want, or expect others to do for them. They might have little to no control over their bodily functions, and may not be able to take care of themselves, or even able to cover their exposed bodies. In this context, their fear of their situation is easier to understand. Likewise, when the caretaker expresses their own vulnerability, it is incredibly meaningful to the patient, and they will be more empathetic to your demanding job.

9. Have only the best of intentions when delivering news and make eye contact.

Good intentions go a long way in creating a positive setting and context for discussions. Even if things don't go as planned, working from high ideals positions you as a truthful and caring person who has others' best interests at heart.

This is where the circumstances of a situation become so important. Patients and family members assume that the medical team will have the best of intentions when delivering news. Depending on the delivery, good or bad news can be difficult to recognize. How are you looking at your patients when you deliver good or bad news? Is your nonverbal communication helping or confusing the situation? Is it possible for you to empathize and say something like, "I know it must be difficult to comprehend all of this information, but I'm happy to answer any questions or concerns you might have, if that helps?" Or, "I'm sorry; I know this was not the news you were expecting or wanted to hear. Can I help you in any way as you process what I've just said?" Knowing that you care and have only the best of intentions in caring for patients as individuals is incredibly meaningful to them and their family members.

10. Set the tone by sticking to the things you know and are relevant to the situation.

Being mindful of the "fire hose" of information that patients are often exposed to, provide only the information that your patients need to know at this particular moment of their treatment. If they have asked you a question, answer that question before adding more information into the mix. Try to resist dominating or taking over a conversation. Refrain from trying to immediately solve the problem or offer a myriad of potential treatments. Be open, curious, and ask questions that confirm the recipient's full understanding. Your ability to set a tone of stability, stating what's relevant in a situation, and also asking follow-up questions, all work to establish closer connections and provide the most relevant dialogue to this situation.

A dear colleague and friend of mine shared with me that when her mom was in the hospital and she was 2000 miles away, she spoke with her mother about results from tests that had just come in. Her mom explained what the results were, but led with what the nurse had said over the phone to her mother. "Well, you don't have cancer..." was what the nurse had said before giving her mom a positive account of her medical status. Sadly, my friend's mom could only focus on the "you don't have cancer" part and continued to question my friend on why the nurse would say that if they were NOT checking for cancer.

Patient Speak

What could be a relief to one person can cause another to obsess over a circumstance that does not even exist when taken out of context (as in this particular situation where cancer was NEVER a concern). Be very careful with your words when speaking to a patient or family member by sticking to what it IS rather than on what it is NOT.

Questions to Ask Your Team

Are we doing our best to alleviate fears of patients and families from the get-go?

Are we consistent in our words as well as our body language and tone of voice when speaking with patients and family members?

Do we have processes in place to deliver consistent communication from the beginning of our interaction with patients and family members?

Are we being considerate of how this information will affect a patient or family member when they are hearing something for the first time?

Patient Speak

Chapter 7

The Fifth C of Communication – Concreteness

"The very first law in advertising is to avoid the concrete promise and cultivate the delightfully vague."

— Stuart Chase, American economist, social theorist, and writer

Concreteness, *adjective.*

1: constituting an actual thing or instance; real:
   "a concrete proof of his sincerity."

2: pertaining to or concerned with realities or actual instances rather than abstractions; particular (as opposed to general): *"concrete ideas."*

3: representing or applied to an actual substance or thing, as opposed to an abstract quality:
   "the words 'cat,' 'water,' and 'teacher' are concrete, whereas the words 'truth,' 'excellence,' and 'adulthood' are abstract."

4: to make real, tangible, or particular.

Patient Speak

As much as being "concrete" in our communication helps people to better understand a concept or condition, the nuance used in the explanation is also essential. Considering the awareness and sensibilities of other people gives them the ability to comprehend, appreciate, and respond to complex yet connected parts.

Using concrete, simple, and easily understood language will always help the receiver to discern messages. As a communicator, ideally you want to speak clearly, yet sensitively. There's an art to speaking concretely with sensitivity, much of which involves tone of voice, as well as nonverbal communication or body language.

In the 1970s, professor of psychology Albert Mehrabian studied the effects of conflicting messages and the importance of nonverbal communication to better understand interpersonal communication. Mehrabian demonstrated in his communication model that only 7% of what we communicate consists of the literal content of a message. The tone and volume of one's voice account for 38%, and as much as 55% of all communication consists of body language. Clearly, the influence of nonverbal communication is stronger than was first assumed.

That is why the spoken word, along with body language (facial expressions, stance, eye contact, etc.), needs to be congruent when communicating with others.

As a medical professional, it's important to pay attention to how the interactions you have with co-workers can affect patients as well. I knew the members of my team that got along well versus ones that did not. I remember being weaned off the ventilator and having someone by my side 24/7 watching the machine bedside. I was in an almost constant state of unrest and panic—feeling that I was suffocating during this transition.

One evening, I was particularly frightened and my nurse was trying to calm me down and had exchanged her dissatisfaction (in my mind) toward the gentleman who was watching the respirator. He walked out and I went into a full-blown panic attack. My room filled with other staff members of the ICU. He never returned and I was just as glad, as I sensed her dissatisfaction with him. However, it is very scary for a patient to witness conflict between members of the medical team. Although I never heard them exchange a word, I could sense in their body language that something was "off." I never saw that particular man again, but I was still concerned about their interaction.

1. Eliminate ambiguity with clear and measured delivery.

To be an effective communicator, you must be equally clear in your tone of voice and body language as you are with the words you choose. When verbal and nonverbal communication are in alignment, ambiguity is erased, and trust is gained. "Measuring" information, that is giving enough to be useful, while not leaving facts and ideas out or letting your patient "guess," help to maintain clarity and trust.

As a member of a medical team, you walk a tightrope in wanting to be honest, forthright, and clear in your communication. At the same time, your "audience" of sick people and those who care for them (friends, family members, etc.) are already in an emotional state of fear, fatigue, and ignorance. Being sensitive to the way you deliver information is very critical.

It is also important to know when to say something versus knowing when it is better to wait to get more answers before sharing information. The best strategy is to ask early on who is going to be the liaison between the medical personnel and the patient (for example, a family member or friend) if the patient is unable to hear complex or challenging news.

2. Distinguish fact from opinion and prioritize discussion points.

Be very clear with your patients whether you are sharing a fact or an opinion. The symptoms are concrete facts and what to do about them is an educated and professional opinion. However, if you have gained your patient's trust, they are likely to take that opinion for fact. Regardless of fact or opinion, prioritize the most important things that need to be conveyed. Know the difference between what you must say now and what you can wait to share after you get more information. Knowing the distinction between what someone must know now and what can wait for later disclosure builds your credibility and increases the trust people have in you.

Always think of how to deliver information to patients—with the most important recommendations that need immediate attention first—and offer a clear explanation as to why they are a priority and the suggested course of treatment. Bring up other points as needed and as they relate to the highest-priority item(s) that need to be addressed. Help patients organize their thoughts based on urgency.

3. Be on time for appointments, meetings, or procedures. Make sure these times are reasonable.

Be respectful of your time and that of others. Show up on time for meetings; be clear when asking someone to be somewhere at a particular time or location and stick to it. If you are not able to do so, give people warning of schedule changes, and as much as possible, adjustments in location and other changes. Not respecting people's time shows a lack of consideration and chips away at the "concreteness" of your credibility.

Patients are far less concerned with having to wait for a doctor or appointment than you might think—assuming we have faith and a connection to our medical team. Having said that, a courtesy call, or update on how long a wait might be would go a long way in a patient's or family member's level of patience. It would be nice to know that someone is running behind and there's time if you need to get something to eat, have lab work done, etc. I know first-hand, and have heard from others that their time is often wasted by waiting when they could be doing other things that also need to be completed to maintain their health.

So often, patients are woken up predawn to be told of a procedure that will "happen soon." Hours later, they are still lying and waiting to be taken to another part of the hospital where the evaluation, test, or procedure will occur. When patients are told of these plans far in advance and incur a loss of sleep, it causes undo stress, anxiety, and fatigue. In business or in other aspects of life, we don't simply ignore a planned meeting that does not take place without explanation.

In hospitals as in most settings, it is understandable that situations can change. But if patients can sleep another hour instead of being woken predawn, forewarned, and then waiting around for hours in advance for a procedure, they will appreciate that. It shows you respect them, and respect leads to trust.

4. Create a quiet setting for effective communication.

For effective communication and understanding to take place, distractions must be kept to a minimum. Removing or reducing background noise, if possible, is key to a better exchange of information and greater understanding. When people have a limited ability to hear, due to their own impairment or to outside interference, clear communication is compromised.

If a patient's hearing is limited, always ask in a polite tone of voice whether he or she hears and understands the information you're presenting.

Patients believe that when equipment is beeping, alarms are going off, or monitors are blinking, something must be critically wrong. They fret that their medications are no longer entering their bodies though their IVs, or there's a malfunction in the equipment that is monitoring their health, and so on. Patients think and envision the worst-case scenarios, and their fear increases with every noise. This is especially true in intensive care units where conscious patients see medical staff racing to other rooms attempting to save the lives of their floor mates. This noise is not only stressful to patients, it can significantly impair clear communication.

5. Offer documentation of discussions at meetings and appointments.

When board meetings occur, there is typically a secretary taking notes of proceedings of what was discussed. These notes remind everyone of the topics covered and inform others who were absent. Without notes it's difficult to remember everything that is discussed during a meeting. The same protocol should be implemented for patient meetings.

Patients and family members appreciate being provided with notes of their meetings with their medical team that they could review, reread, and think about after the medical team has left the room. Thankfully, Tom Delbanco, MD and Jan Walker of Beth Israel Deaconess Medical Center in Boston created OpenNotes that many hospitals use. Patients can look at the digital notes on their medical records online and communicate with their doctors to correct information, clarify comments, and have full access to their doctors' "voices" about their condition.

Offering a patient a written protocol about their course of treatment, or any other information that is exchanged, is a helpful reference, and might also encourage greater adherence to medical advice. Frustration levels on all sides will also decrease when there are written instructions and information about people's medical conditions and treatments that are easily accessible to all parties.

6. Summarize key points of a conversation.

Similar to notes of a meeting, offering a one-page summary of key points with action items can provide participants a to-do list of attainable next actions.

Provide patients with guidelines written in plain language and including patient-friendly tools, such as medical illustrations of anatomy, suggested questions for doctors, and a glossary of terms, tests, and treatment options. Offering patients objective, expert guidance allows them to better understand and discuss their illness and treatment options with their providers.

7. Never lie or mislead someone into believing something that is untrue.

Intentionally misleading or deceiving someone is wrong. Omitting, concealing, or falsifying information is equivalent to lying. Verbal or written deceit tactics involve fabrication, distortion, evasiveness, non-responsiveness, and denial.

In medicine, it's particularly important to be transparent, especially when complications arise, and talk of things that are concrete. Never minimize problems, fail to tell the whole truth, or resort to oversimplifying situations. It's never easy to deliver sad news or admit to a lapse of judgment or medical error. However, being forthcoming and honest can reduce potential lawsuits. After all, medical professionals are human and can make mistakes, too. Being honest and admitting the truth earns you trust and validity in the important work you do.

8. Speak plainly.

Have you ever visited a country where you didn't speak the language, and the only word you knew was "toilet?" That's often how patients feel when their caretakers use medical jargon. It may seem to show that you know what you're talking about, but is more likely to have the opposite effect, distancing you from your patient and peers. Keep your language simple and clear for the highest level of understanding and connection.

Patients and their families are often overwhelmed when listening to instructions for care, diagnoses, and treatment plans. Speaking any kind of vernacular will lead to confusion for one simple reason: patients haven't learned a language or studied and practiced the way medical professionals have. Ask if your patients understood what you have said and see if they have any questions about what you have explained to them. Chances are they do.

Encourage them to write down questions that might occur to them later if none come to mind at the moment. Keeping conversations straightforward will lessen turmoil and confusion.

9. Deliver a series of actions designed to deliver desired results.

Results are achieved by focusing on the behaviors and actions that generate them. The benefit of detailed steps and protocols systematize communication procedures to achieve a consistent result in every interaction.

As in the earlier example of the role-playing exercise of an intern who was doing an intake in ICU with her patient, providing context would have been helpful to reduce the patient's fear and anxiety. If a particular protocol or method was designed to do intakes consistently, the results— understanding end-of-life issues and naming a healthcare proxy—would be achieved without alarming or upsetting the patient. A concrete list of questions in a specific order, with the patient in mind, will achieve the desired results in a compassionate and caring manner.

10. Have as many face-to-face interactions as possible.

We live in a digital world, and that is a good thing for many reasons. Information is transmitted and available immediately; our ability to communicate, monitor, and oversee important items and issues allows us to be more connected than ever before. However, there remains no true replacement for face-to-face communication, where a complete and concrete interaction can only be achieved by experiencing someone's facial expressions, tone of voice, and body language. Although it's not always possible, in an ideal world, this is the most effective way to deliver sensitive news, advice, or instructions.

Seeing a doctor or nurse who can deliver crucial or sensitive material or advice, face-to-face, is always preferred. It allows for having concerns and questions to be asked and answered immediately. The Society of Participatory Medicine was created to bring together physicians and patients to become more engaged as partners in medical care. This places a greater emphasis and demand on the relationship between doctor and patient and on an open and honest exchange of concrete information between them.

Questions to Ask Your Team

Are we working effectively to eliminate co-worker conflict and ensure our patients do not witness personality conflicts while in our care?

Are we working to simplify language and be clear with what we want our patients and family members to know about their case?

Are we working to ensure that patient's time is being respected, and that we are communicating with them when there are delays or interruptions with appointment times, etc.?

Do we do our best in letting patients or family members know when we will be making rounds, or be available to speak on the phone to answer additional questions they may have?

Patient Speak

Chapter 8

The Sixth C of Communication – Courtesy or Consideration

"Being considerate of others will take your children further in life than any college degree."

— Marian Wright Edelman, American children's activist

Courtesy, *noun, plural,* courtesies.

1: excellence of manners or social conduct; polite behavior.

2: a courteous, respectful, or considerate act or expression.

Consideration, *noun.*

1: the act of considering; careful thought; meditation; deliberation: *"I will give your project full consideration."*

2: something that is or is to be kept in mind in making a decision, evaluating facts, etc.: *"age was an important consideration in the decision."*

3: thoughtful or sympathetic regard or respect; thoughtfulness for others: *"they showed no consideration for his feeling."*

4: a thought or reflection; an opinion based upon reflection.

Patient Speak

Chapter 8: Courtesy or Consideration

Being *courteous* is a relatively simple concept: Treat others as you would like to be treated. A feeling of goodwill is generated between people who show respect and consideration for others. Courtesy must be sincere and genuine to be believable. Having and demonstrating good manners is also a way of showing civility and kindness. When we exhibit these qualities, we draw people to us and make them feel welcomed and comfortable. When treated with courtesy and consideration, patients feel valued and good about themselves.

Patients and family members seek hospitals, doctors and specialists most often by referrals from our primary care physician, friends, or family members who we know, like and trust. We feel confident that if someone is being recommended, then they have been vetted and are deemed trustworthy, competent and well-respected. We all want the best and most qualified person to treat us or a loved one—the best person for the job of helping us heal.

I am so grateful that my primary care physician made the referral to my medical team after receiving my lab work from my local ER. I am also grateful for his visits while I was hospitalized and his concerned follow up of my case. It was a professional courtesy to refer my doctor, but it was a life or death situation for me as well.

1. Act in the best interest of others.

Having another person's best interest at heart and acting in that manner lends itself to greater trust. Acting in the best interest of people shows them that you care for their well-being.

In medicine, the credo "do no harm" speaks to the intent of all medical professionals. When patients and family members first learn about their condition and the course of treatment, consider that the news may be shocking, scary, and unthinkable. Remind them that you know this might be very difficult to hear, but you have their best interests at heart and will take good care of them.

Sensitivity to others' feelings, especially when they are receiving potentially devastating news, speaks volumes about your humanity and desire to look out for their best options and outcomes. Patients and their family members respect medical professionals who can deliver a message with awareness and sensitivity. Sharing that you are acting in their best interests with the course of action you're recommending instills belief and confidence in you and your work.

2. Strive for open and honest communication.

Showing respect and civility goes hand-in-hand with communication that is forthright, considerate, and honest. Deception of any kind breaks down the trust in relationships and can result in irreparable damage.

In medical situations, a lack of open and honest communication leads your patients to believe that you may be hiding something. It's never easy to deal with a mistake that might have been made or an incorrect diagnosis; however, being honest about what happened and offering a solution to help solve the problem in the future goes a long way in solidifying a relationship. We are all human and we all make mistakes. It's how we deal with those mistakes that shows our true character. Take responsibility. When something goes wrong, take responsibility and own your mistakes. Patients trust people who are responsible.

3. Speak directly to the person you're talking to and be aware of nonverbal communication.

Making eye contact and looking directly at the person or people you are talking to are essential to good communication. People better understand what is being said when you look them in the eye.

Patients often may be hard of hearing or dependent on an interpreter or parent/guardian to understand what is being said. They may be too young or too elderly to fully understand what is being said. It's very important to look directly at both the patient and the person who may be helping to translate or explain what you are saying. Good communication is essential, so patients understand critical details about medications, surgeries, procedures, and aftercare. It's also important to be aware of patients who have any hearing difficulties and to be sure to have their attention before you begin talking to them.

Here are some ways you can be more effective when talking to your patients:

- *Face patients when talking to them*
- *Slow the rate of speech so there is space between words*
- *Speak clearly*
- *Make eye contact*
- *Smile*
- *Use a caring tone of voice*
- *Speak with positive affirmation*
- *Nod your head when you understand*
- *Respect your patients' choices*
- *Treat your patients like equals*
- *Stay calm in emergencies*

4. Ask questions and listen carefully.

When you take the time to truly listen, it shows you value the other person's perspective and life experience. Whomever you are listening to will feel good when they realize you are hearing them and attempting to understand what they are saying. Explicitly asking questions shows the other person that you value his or her opinion, and you will get answers that will help you to better comprehend where the person is coming from. Try not to interrupt someone who is talking; interrupting is similar to showing up late. It sends a message that what you have to say is more important than what anyone else has to say, or that your time is more important than theirs. Listen instead; listening shows respect for the other person's point of view. The person who knows how to listen is the person who will always be trusted. Be understanding. Seek first to understand, and then to be understood.

Many times, patients or family members won't ask you questions initially. You have to understand that this is the first time they are hearing the information you are presenting, even though you've delivered it several times to many people. Patients are "virgins" of the message or news you are delivering. Be gentle with them. When your patients have something to say, allow them time to complete their thoughts, and then respond with empathy and compassion. Hearing patients out when they are able to speak, ask questions, and inquire about their specific situations will go a long way in establishing a long-term relationship based on trust.

Always listen to your patients. If they have a health issue or complaint, then listening helps you to understand and comfort them appropriately. Listening will allow you to pick up on symptoms or feelings that patients may not be aware of or don't know how to express. Ask them questions about their physical and emotional needs as well as caregiving preferences. If they want to be served meals a certain way, accommodate them if possible. Acting on their requests can immensely improve their frame of mind and physical condition.

5. Use touch appropriately.

A gentle touch goes a long way. To be sure touch is welcome, ask first. Try, "Would you like a hug?" or "May I touch your shoulder?" Gentle touch assists in balancing physical, mental, emotional, and spiritual well-being. A soft touch to the hand or shoulder during the conversation helps demonstrate a genuine care and concern for the other person.

https://www.nancymichaels.com/single-post/2018/08/06/ From-ICU-to-I-See-You

When thinking about touching a patient, situations may vary greatly. A recent topic of discussion came up in a PFAC (Patient Family Advisory Council) discussion on Facebook, "To Hug or Not?" The conversation was framed with a story about a physician whose human instinct tells him to offer a hug to his patients when they become upset, but in the current cultural climate, he has found himself holding back, unsure of what the patient wants and needs in that situation and what the perception might be if he offers a hug.

A panel of medical, spiritual, and patient relation representatives offered their perspectives on medical professionals offering hugs to—or not hugging—patients who become emotional. There's no easy answer for this because most people find physical contact between doctors and nurses and their patients more or less acceptable.

The PFAC asked the patients attending the session how they might respond after receiving upsetting information from their or their family member's doctor that makes them emotional. *"Under what circumstances, if any, would it be okay for the doctor to comfort you with a hug? What might you say to a classroom full of doctors-in-training about 'the right way' to comfort a patient when a patient becomes emotional?"*

A co-PFAC patient member responded with this statement. "I have several doctors that start and end visits with hugs. They read me, they know I accept them. I've been hugged by my oncologist I've known for fifteen years. But recently, a radiology tech (whom I had never met before) ended a very recent (session where I had a) biopsy with a hug. Both (hugs) were welcomed and comforting. On the other hand, there are several doctors I have that, if they offered a hug, (the hugs) would not be comforting. It's mostly about the connection between two people. There is no easy answer or black-and-white formula. While we can't easily explain or teach body language, I would start there. It's a fine line, isn't it? Offering what feels like natural comfort (which may be received as such) versus initiating potentially threatening behavior."

In the end, her advice was to err on the side of caution, and she suggested that the preferred behavior in dealing with most patients would be not to offer physical contact. This is a tricky one. It might be welcome for a doctor, nurse, physical therapist, etc. to ask a patient if it's ok to give them a hug or a pat on the back to gauge their level of comfort or discomfort with the act.

Personally, as a patient, I feel very connected to my medical team and would in no way be put off by personal contact, but I realize I may not be the norm. I do remember more than a year ago, when I was told I needed to have both hips replaced (eventually), but one hip replacement was imminent, feeling very upset and confused. When I met for my six-month checkup with my liver doctor (who didn't make this diagnosis, but knew of it), he sat on a small rolling chair and came very close to me and took both of my hands and looked into my eyes and said, "Nancy, this should NOT have happened to you. You were on very low doses of prednisone (I had two organ rejections early on after my liver transplant). We just don't see this happening to people like you that often." I became more emotional but so appreciated his warmth, concern, and compassion. I also feel that people will either tell you they're not comfortable with physical contact or you can sense it right away in their body language and how they respond. It's not a cookie-cutter situation, and caretakers probably should take the patient's personality, demeanor, culture, ethnicity, and so on into consideration in each situation.

6. Be honest and ask for honesty in return.

Honest communication breeds trust. Honesty is truly the best policy. You cannot expect that people will be honest with you if they sense you are not being honest with them.

Clinicians realize that making accurate diagnoses depends on the reliability of the information provided by patients and their family members. Sharing with patients and family members that you will always be forthright and honest with them is important. Likewise, it's essential you let them know that you also expect honesty from them as well. Honest, effective communication allows for astute, timely, and compassionate care and depends on the truthful relationship between patients and physicians.

7. Remember and use the name of the person you are addressing.

Courteous people use the name of the people they are addressing. You can always ask the people you're talking to what they prefer to be called (nickname, more formal salutation, etc.) because it's considerate to address people that way. The important thing is to address them by their name; you can learn their preferred name later.

Patients and family members very much appreciate your addressing them by their name. It reinforces the personal nature of what you do by acknowledging them in this way. It sends a message to them that they know you care because you know who they are as human beings, that you are paying attention, and that you care about them and their feelings, which leads to greater trust.

8. Be considerate of the people you are communicating with and about what is important to them.

Honesty is important but understanding where the person you are addressing is coming from is also imperative. As a human being, your patient has feelings, and being "honest to a fault" is not helpful to a relationship. Not everything that is on your mind needs to be expressed truthfully to another person. It takes finesse to know what is appropriate to say to someone versus what can wait to be said later or not at all.

In medicine, clinicians have viewed the withholding of information as essential, if not an obligation, in communicating with patients or family members. Doctors must consider what a patient is ready to hear versus what the absolute truth is. All of the following influence the sharing of information: the patient's condition, the patient's expectations, the seriousness of the condition or illness, and the need for privacy. Subsequently, the type of information a patient is given will make a difference in his or her attitude about the sickness, treatment plan, and overall well-being. Never forget the importance of providing hope to a patient. I strongly believe that the emotional and mental health of a patient contributes significantly to their ability to heal.

9. Be approachable and courteous.

When you are open, available, and approachable, you attract people to you.

Patients and families yearn to approach you and for you to be approachable. Patients appreciate more than you know that your expertise and knowledge of their condition is far greater than their own, and that you are available to them. As a courteous person, you never flaunt your expert "status," but instead you always make your patients feel important. As Albert Mehrabian suggests, your body language sends clear signals about your approachability as well. Lean in when speaking to your patients; smile at them and act as if you are as honored to know them as they are to know and be treated by you.

10. Address the difficult and unpleasant with empathy and grace.

It is human nature to not want to contemplate or discuss obvious problems and difficult situations. We avoid talking about things that concern or bother us for our own sake and the sake of others. Ignoring the "elephant in the room" is never the best approach, because in the end, we need to address challenging cases regardless of how difficult they are. Ignoring a potentially unpleasant condition does not make it go away.

Patient Speak

It may seem easy to avoid the inevitable, but in the end, patients and family members need to know what to expect and understand their options and ability to make choices about how they want to continue to live their lives. This is especially true in end-of-life scenarios when people need to make difficult choices. The most compassionate thing a caregiver can do in this situation is to be open to discussing all available options with kindness and consideration of all parties involved.

Questions to Ask Your Team

How are we showing our sincere interest in our patients?

What are some of the ways we can attempt to put ourselves in their shoes?

Are we able to admit mistakes and apologize?

Are we aware of our body language when speaking to patients or family members?

Do we appear rushed or short with them? How can we slow down and take the time to hear them out?

Patient Speak

Chapter 9

The Seventh C of Communication – Compassion

"Love and compassion are necessities, not luxuries. Without them humanity cannot survive."

— Dalai Lama, Spiritual Leader of the Tibetan People

Compassion, *noun.*

1: a feeling of deep sympathy and sorrow for another who is stricken by misfortune, accompanied by a strong desire to alleviate the suffering.

Patient Speak

Compassion is having a genuine feeling of empathy for someone's hardship or suffering, with a desire to alleviate his or her pain. Ideally, compassion is heartfelt and sincere. Empathy is the ability to put yourself in someone else's shoes. Your empathy and compassion deepen all relationships, and there are many ways to demonstrate it.

I'm fortunate to have a very compassionate team who have been treating me for the past 13 years. They have taken the time to hear my concerns about a doctor (not mine) I wasn't pleased with, gave me hope when I needed it, and delivered news clearly but with compassion.

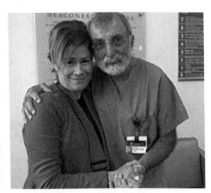

Me and Frank in 2016, 11 years after my transplant

One act of compassion and kindness I'll never forget is when my nurse Frank had seen me mouth out (I had a trachea) my desire to go outside. It was August, and I had recently awoken from a two-month-long coma. Doctors repeatedly said I was too immune-suppressed after undergoing an emergency liver transplant. One day, Frank arrived prior to his shift and offered to take me to a CT scan. After I left radiology, he took me down a hallway that was unfamiliar to me and through two large black double doors onto the loading zone of the hospital. Frank pushed the gurney into the sun and lifted the blanket off my legs. He stood silently by my side for about five minutes before returning me to the ICU.

I have not stopped telling audiences and now readers about the compassion Frank offered me by performing this simple act of kindness and compassion.

Article "Perfectly Frank": *https://www.nancymichaels.com/single-post/2018/08/14/Perfectly-Frank*

1. Practice the habit of being empathic.

There is perhaps no better way to show compassion than to empathize, and show you understand what your patients are going through. If you want people to hear you, offer them empathy and understanding before you offer advice or potential solutions. Emotional intelligence, the capacity to be aware of, control, and express your emotions, and to handle interpersonal relationships judiciously and empathetically, allows you to acknowledge the feelings of others and act accordingly. Your communication is easier when your patients feel you understand them.

Being able to understand and empathize with your patients is key to establishing a trusting relationship. Acknowledging and respecting patients' concerns, desires, or points of view makes them feel better cared for and justified in their opinions about their health and well-being. They feel they can communicate more openly and clearly with you. You are better able to deliver the best care possible when trust and understanding have been established with your patients.

2. Be calm and clear in your communication.

Very few if any people admire an alarmist style of communication. It's discourteous to speak loudly, yell, or overdramatize a topic you want to have a productive conversation about. An overzealous reaction or discussion of a topic can shut down or eliminate a chance to effectively communicate. It can be considered rude and unproductive.

Patients are very sensitive to noises or strained conversations they overhear on the hospital floor or tension between medical staff. Respect is given when people perform their medical duties calmly and with respect to their coworkers. When patients sense unease among their medical team or hear discordant discourse, they are affected by it and might begin to question the care they are being given. I gave an example of this when I was in ICU and getting off of the respirator in the previous chapter.

3. Show appreciation and awareness of spatial surroundings.

Being conscious of someone's environment is important when wanting to communicate with compassion. The concept of spatial awareness is, in this sense, to be in tune with what is happening around you in the moment. When you are perceptive of the situation, the people involved, and the priorities, you show respect, consideration, and compassion for the person you are communicating with, and any other people who are present.

A patient was having her hair washed by a kind nurse who knew the patient's children were coming to see her the following day, and she wanted to make this patient feel and look good. While washing the patient's hair, the nurse began talking with her assistant about the ongoing discussion she and her husband were having about whether or not to have a third child. The patient started crying because she hadn't seen her three children in months and was hurt by the personal conversation between the two nurses who were taking care of her. Some communication should not take place in front of a patient, especially if it is unrelated to the patient. Although the nurse had the best of intentions, the conversation tainted the kind act of washing the patient's hair in anticipation of her children's visit.

4. Never underestimate the power of offering hope and a second chance whenever reasonably possible.

When people are encouraged and offered positive reinforcement, it can oftentimes generate a renewed, confident series of behaviors and beliefs within them. There is virtually no down side to being positive. This is especially true of people who believe they will not get better or might even be dying.

As much as patients and family members want to be spoken to truthfully, they often want to have a ray of hope in dealing with a medical calamity. Miracles can and do happen. The power of your words as a doctor or nurse are critical to patients' mental and emotional states. Never underestimate the power of the mind to help bodies and spirits heal. Think of how you or a family member would want to be spoken to before receiving a dismal diagnosis. There are exceptions when death is inevitable, but choose your words and how you say them carefully and kindly. Many people are alive and well today (myself included!) when the odds were stacked against them. More focus and belief on the psychological component of healing are essential.

5. Perform small acts of kindness and compassion.

No act of kindness or compassion, however small, is ever wasted. Even if no one else sees it, it will matter to someone and make your heart feel the love you offered.

Pay attention to what might matter to people, and if possible, give it to them without being asked or expecting something in return. A key factor in developing compassion is to give without the assumption that your generosity will be returned.

6. Respect the dignity of others.

Human decency should be shown at all times when communicating with one another. It is never respectful, considerate, or compassionate to speak to people in a way that strips them of their pride or dignity. Patients are human beings and should be treated as such.

Patients are subjected to their personal privacy being invaded or even nonexistent at times. Oftentimes, they have no control over bodily functions and have been reduced from being productive, independent people to being totally reliant on others for almost everything. To say it's demoralizing would be an understatement. Please protect their dignity. Close the door, pull the curtain, and show your respect. Be compassionate and acknowledge that this cannot be easy for them. Be open to listening or offering a different way of interacting that might be helpful.

7. Make an effort to get to know and interact with people on a more personal level.

It may not be easy for everyone to reach out to people and be naturally social; however, few of us can avoid interpersonal communication for long. To show compassion you must be in contact with people and understand where they're coming from, their experiences and emotions.

Getting to know your patients can help you empathize with them better and allow them to feel more comfortable with you. It may also help your patients feel more relaxed when you're assisting them with personal hygiene routines like bathing or feeding. This type of socializing with your patients can occur while you are in their room performing other duties by simply asking them how they're feeling or if they need anything to feel more comfortable. Do this every day. Sometimes patients in long-term-care facilities don't have family members nearby whom they can socialize with.

Take a moment to chat with your patients about their day. If you have time, maybe you can even spend some quality time with them. Try reading a book or watching TV with them while you feed them.

8. Be human.

We are all human, and although patients entrust their health and well-being to their medical team, most reasonable people understand that doctors, nurses, and medical specialists are all human as well and can make mistakes. The best way to avoid unnecessary litigation when a misstep or gaffe occurs is to be open and honest with your communication and admit the lapse in judgment or calculation, and this starts with compassion for yourself.

There is always a way or an opportunity to do things better; that is part of the human experience. Having compassion for yourself in that learning moment is just as important as having compassion for your patients, coworkers and their families.

Additionally, an open, transparent and compassionate communication with patients and their families decreases the chance of lawsuits because patients feel they have a relationship that they value with you. According to the article "Four Ways to Reduce Your Malpractice Risks in Physician's Practice" published on PhysiciansPractice.com, each suggestion was related to communication tactics, including: (1) asking staff to prioritize, (2) increasing physician communication, (3) asking staff to step up, and (4) creating and implementing policies and procedures. Effective communication and compassionate care can overcome your learning moments in a vast majority of instances.

9. Express yourself.

Even though you're dealing with someone else's strong emotions, your own emotions have a place in the interaction.

Match your facial expressions to your emotions to let other people know you understand what they are going through. A sincere smile often works wonders. It is also okay to show sadness and concern. Likewise, a good laugh can be incredibly healing.

10. Be mindful of your words.

Think before you speak. At its heart, *compassion* is about paying attention to the moment you are experiencing with your patients, and being present with a loving and kind attitude. Being present means doing simple things like turning off your cell phone during a personal conversation, asking questions that you're genuinely interested in hearing the responses to, and other like ways of giving them your undivided, genuinely interested attention.

It's easy for anyone to go on and on about something they feel passionate about. We all know things. Cool things. Great things. Just make sure you share those things in the right settings. If you're a mentor, share away. If you're a coach or a leader, share away. If you're the guy who just started a new workout diet plan, refrain from telling your patients what to order unless they ask. Courteous and compassionate people know that what is right for them might not be right for others, and even if it is right, it is not their place to decide that for others. Courteous and compassionate people are always charming.

Courteous and compassionate people are fluent in getting people to talk about themselves without even being aware of it. They are fascinated by you, your life, your family and your aspirations. This happens by asking the right open-ended questions. As soon as you learn a little about someone, ask an obvious follow-up question. Compassion comes when you relate to people on a human level and they relate to you because you're willing to listen. Patients feel heard and understood when you take the time and interest in them.

Asking other people about themselves implicitly shows you respect them. Respect is a form of grace and courtesy. **Never stop being compassionate.**

Patient Speak

Questions to Ask Your Team

What are some of the ways we show compassion to our patients?

Could we do a better job in offering small acts of kindness and compassion to patients and families?

How so?

Are we aware of our conversations in front of patients and what impact they may have on them?

How can we relate on a more human level to our patients and family members who are under tremendous pressure, fatigue and ill health?

Can we do more and how so?

Chapter 9: Compassion

Patient Speak

Conclusion

Genshai and the Positive Effects of Compassionate Communication

In 2006, I was interviewed by a local Fox affiliate where my college friend was a producer of the morning show, and the anchor was also in my graduating class at Emerson College. My friend Carol had pitched the idea of featuring me on the show as a feel good, comeback kind of story. At the time, I was still very much in recovery mode as you could see in my frail physical appearance and my hair still growing in post brain surgery. I had actually asked my nurse to cut off all my hair as opposed to just letting the right side of my hair grow in.

When I was being interviewed, I mentioned a short list of things I had learned when I was sick and in the hospital, and one of them was to do unto others as you would have them do unto you. I meant that then and I still do.

At the beginning of 2012, I launched the New Year by attending a Genshai Mastery Retreat in Coronado, California at the invitation of my dear friend Kristin Andress. Each presenter had the most amazing life stories, ranging from a woman who was held against her will in a polygamous community and risked her life escaping the compound, to another woman who holed up in a bathroom with several other women during the Rwandan genocide against the Tutsi, during which she lost every member of her family. Devastating and immense loss was described by so many men and women who emerged as triumphant spirits despite all odds. This provided heartwarming evidence of the will to live and overcome trauma and tragedy.

The retreat featured Kevin Hall, author of *Aspire: Discovering Your Purpose through the Power of Words*, who shared a story of a secret word he discovered, "Genshai," an ancient Hindi word that means "Never treat others, or yourself, in a way to make them feel small." Kevin spoke of travelling to Vienna, Austria where he met a man there who invited him to sign the *Book of Greats*. This man explained that the *Book of Greats* had been signed by Mother Teresa, Victor Frankel, and many of Gandhi's family members, and others we would consider great. Kevin said that he thought he was not worthy to sign the book, and that's when he was made aware of and understood the meaning of Genshai—that we are all great. At the end of the Genshai retreat, each of us was offered the opportunity to sign the *Book of Greats*. I've reflected on the concept of Genshai many times. When those negative self-talk statements creep into my mind, I remind myself the meaning of Genshai, "to never treat others, or yourself, in a way to make them or you feel small." Ultimately, the spirit of

Genshai is to treat others with respect and honor. It's about having compassion for yourself and those around you.

Isn't that also one of the key objectives in medicine? In addition to helping a person's body to heal, the way we communicate with one another has a significant impact on a person's psyche, and I believe, based on my own experience as a long-term patient, on our ability to help heal ourselves. Words, tone of voice, and body language, all contribute to eliciting emotions from your patients. True compassion comes as a result of having awareness and empathy for another person. It is characterized by kind thoughts, feelings, actions, and words. The simple act of showing compassion can turn someone's day around. There's no need to wait for a crisis situation to practice the art of Genshai, or compassion. Don't believe me? Then try smiling at a stranger today.

https://genshai.com/

It all goes back to one of the four cofounders of Johns Hopkins Hospital, Canadian physician Sir William Osler, who was the first to bring medical students out of the lecture hall for face-to-face bedside training with patients. He also offered an admonition to doctors in the later part of the nineteenth century: to "care more particularly for the individual patient than for the special features of the disease."

Dr. Francis Weld Peabody was an American physician from Cambridge, Massachusetts and one of the most quoted professors at Harvard Medical School. He famously reiterated the subject of compassion in his frequently quoted remark to the graduating class at Harvard in 1926: "Time, sympathy, and understanding must be lavishly dispensed, but the reward is to be found in that personal bond which forms the greatest satisfaction of the practice of medicine. One of the essential qualities of the clinician is interest in humanity, for the secret of the care of the patient is in caring for the patient."

In 2011, the year of his death, Dr. J. Willis Hurst, the cardiologist for Lyndon B. Johnson from the time of his first heart attack in 1955, and the principal editor of *The Heart*, hosted interns and residents at his retirement home for a monthly lecture. He introduced them to Dr. Francis W. Peabody by reading the statement above. He then asked, "*Why* should patients know that their doctor cares about them?"

After discussing the issue, the young doctors came to the conclusion that when patients know that their doctor cares about them as people, it helps create a bond of trust, which improves compliance. When compliance improves, the patient improves. The best way to show patients how much you care is to communicate with them in a manner that demonstrates your interest and concern for them as human beings.

Conclusion

Patient Speak

To My Readers

Let's continue the conversation – here's how...

I'm hoping you enjoyed this book and have gained a new perspective by seeing communication through the lens of the patient.

Just as telemedicine, digital health, and mobile technology are impacting healthcare, the publishing industry has adapted to online and on-demand sales, "reading" or listening to books, and, of course, how books are reviewed. Thank you Amazon! I thank you in advance if you'd like to review *Patient Speak* online.

I'm also wondering how we might work together to create more win-win relationships—a win for you as a healthcare professional who's admired by patients and families for your exceptional ability to show warmth, encouragement, and openness in your professional liaisons—and a win for the patients you have devoted your life to serve and help heal.

My talks are always customized to my audience, and I would be honored to create a custom book for you. We can tailor-make these handbooks to suit your brand and purpose—from adding your logo and affiliations to the cover, to altering the examples to suit your specific industry. Order your custom booklet direct in bulk to receive a competitive price per unit.

Please e-mail Team@NancyMichaels.com, to arrange a time to talk and iron out the details.

About the Author

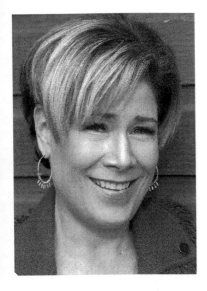

Nancy Michaels works with organizations to provide VIP customer engagement within healthcare, medical and retail organizations who want to ensure the lifetime loyalty of their consumer base. She speaks on ways to improve the overall experience, retention and referrals through more effective communication and trust building strategies.

She offers a generously poignant perspective on her collective life experiences – beginning with her career as a public speaker and business development consultant . . . turned patient. In 2005, Nancy found herself in a health crisis that would nearly twice end her life. In that year, Nancy underwent an emergent liver transplant and brain surgery that brought with them significant medical complications and left her in a two-month coma. Waking up was a blessing; working to overcome the fallout of her ordeal was a battle.

NANCY MICHAELS
Healthcare Speaker, Inspirational Speaker, Consultant

Nancy hopes you stay in touch.

- You can read her thoughts, tirades, and tactics on Twitter: www.twitter.com/NancyMichaels

- Associate for business networking on LinkedIn: www.linkedin.com/in/nmichaels

- Acquire free training, announcements, and posts on Facebook: www.facebook.com/nancymichaelsfans

- Visit Nancy's website—www.NancyMichaels.com—to download her *10 Lessons Learned from Dying*, sign up for her monthly newsletter *Speaking of Patient Satisfaction*, and read her blog.

To book Nancy for your next conference or event, contact Team@NancyMichaels.com

Patient Speak

Bibliography

Bailey, Melissa. "Medical Schools Incorporate Arts into
   Doctors' Training." *STAT*, 20 July 2016,
   www.statnews.com/2015/11/03/why-medical-schools-
   are-adding-courses-in-literature-and-dance/.

Brooks, Andrew A. "Going from Good to Great Care –
   5 Ways to Boost HCAHPS Scores." *Becker's Hospital
   Review*, 7 Apr. 2014, www.beckershospitalreview.com/
   quality/going-from-good-to-great-care-5-ways-to-boost-
   hcahps-scores.html.

Patient Speak

Resources

Although the topic of patient and family satisfaction, experience and engagement is gaining ground and resources are growing, here are a few that might benefit the reader to have access to.

Some are topics that are relevant to improving the patient experience and others are friends and colleagues of mine who are working alongside me toward this end.

I hope you enjoy and can benefit from knowing about them and reading, watching or listening to what they might offer on this important topic.

Patient Family Advisory Councils

Forming a Patient and Family Advisory Council | STEPS Forward

https://www.stepsforward.org/modules/pfac

by MJ Hatlie – Related articles

Aug 31, 2016 – Eight STEPS to form and get to work with your patient (or person) and family advisory council **(PFAC) Develop** your practice's business case for the **PFAC** and ensure leadership support. **Create a PFAC** planning committee. Develop an action plan, charter and budget. Invite, interview and select **PFAC** members.

Kistein Monkhouse, MPA is a friend and colleague of mine who was a nursing assistant by trait for several years. She is a public health administrator by education turned videographer and advocate for family members, caretakers and nurses who have huge knowledge of patients' unique circumstances and needs. She's turned her passion for caring for the ill into a traveling documentary of public opinion about our healthcare system. Some of the participants speak on the overall healthcare environment and others share their patient experience as well.

Civic Engagements: Thoughts On U.S Healthcare System
https://www.patientorator.com/video-blog/civic-engagements

Article featuring two doctors at Cooper University Hospital who are fearful of the lack of compassion in healthcare.

http://www.philly.com/archive/stacey_burling/cooper-doctors-study-compassion-crisis-in-health-care-20180315.html

Compassion, Doc Communication Create Positive Patient Experience

An analysis of Healthgrades surveys shows that patient experience scores improve when providers deliver compassionate care with good communication.

https://www.beckershospitalreview.com/quality/going-from-good-to-great-care-5-ways-to-boost-hcahps-scores.html

My friend, colleague and sometimes co-presenter, **Danny van Leeuwen, MPH, RN, CPHQ**, is a nationally recognized nurse leader and advocate for family caregivers. He's an ePatient with multiple sclerosis, a caregiver, a nurse, and a leader. He has led the Patient Family Experience initiative for Boston Children's Hospital, serves on the HIMSS Connected Patients Committee, and is a member of the Society for Participatory Medicine. He speaks nationally about family caregivers and health information technology and hosts a weekly blog (http://www.health-hats.com) with more than 2,000 registered users. His career includes experience as a nurse, QI director, health informatics specialist, author, and researcher. He attained national recognition for his published works in the Joint Commission Journal on Quality Safety and the Journal for Healthcare Quality, where he was an editor for 15 years.

https://www.health-hats.com/trust/

Another dear friend and colleague, **Susan Baker**, does an exceptional job of reviewing a few articles each week that relate to customer and patient care and service. Learn more at www.susanbaker.com.

The Society for Participatory Medicine is a 501(c)(3) not-for-profit organization devoted to promoting the concept of participatory medicine, a movement in which networked patients shift from being mere passengers to responsible drivers of their health, and in which providers encourage and value them as full partners. The Society seeks to bring together all of the stakeholders in healthcare (patients, caregivers, healthcare professionals, payers, and others) to encourage collaboration, communication and cooperation that will foster provider/patient engagement, patient empowerment and education.

Report – Clinical Communication Deconstructed 2017. pdf
https://www.psqh.com/resource/clinical-communication-deconstructed-seven-elements-effective-clinical-communication/